SAFE SEX

a guide to condoms

Second Edition

By
James W. Brackett
International Population Specialist

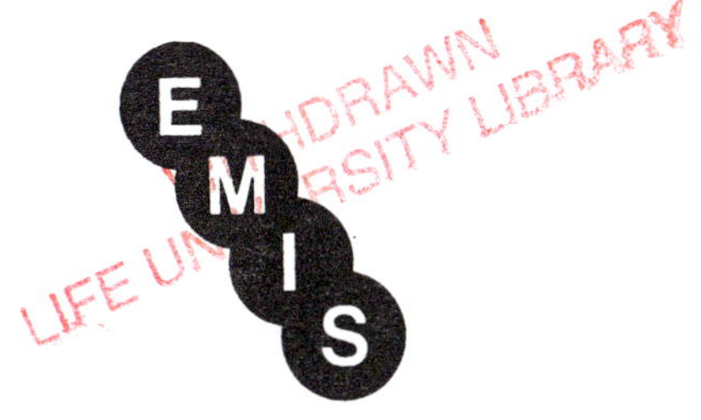

Essential Medical
Information Systems, Inc.
P. O. Box 1607
Durant, OK 74702
1-800-225-0694

For Direct Mail Orders:

**Essential Medical
Information Systems, Inc.**
P.O. Box 1607
Durant, OK 74702

Telephone Orders:

1-800-225-0694

SECOND EDITION
Published in the United States 1991

ISBN:
0-929240-25-1

Printed in the United States of America

Acknowledgments

A number of individuals deserve special mention for their assistance during the writing of this book.

First, to my wife, Maura Brackett, who served as critic and editor as well as a continuing source of inspiration and patience.

To her sister, Lea Gill, who collected price data in the Hartford area.

To my son, Nathaniel Brackett and his wife, Sue who collected price data in the Pittsburgh area.

To Hank Lawrence, who collected price data in the San Francisco area.

And finally, to Dr. John Wells, who commissioned me to write a book on condoms and provided continuing support and outstanding style and content guidance.

CENTER INDEX SYSTEM

The purpose of the center index system is to enable readers to immediately locate all the information contained in the book. Tabs are provided with each center index so there is a direct connection between the center index and text. The text is organized in a sequential format to enable the reader to proceed to any area of the text without having to read through information not relevant to the situation.

TABLE OF CONTENTS

TABLES

FIGURE

#1 Overview

Condoms are "prophylactics," or preventive devices. They have two purposes: to reduce the risk of sexually transmitted disease (STD) and to reduce the risk of unwanted pregnancy.

There are historical records dating back more than 3,000 years of men wearing sheaths over the glans of their penises, but history has not revealed the purpose of these sheaths.

By the 18th century, European meat processing workmen had a lively trade selling animal intestine, or "skins," for use as condoms. These "skins" were clearly intended to be used during sexual intercourse to protect against STDs and pregnancy.

Prostitutes, apparently the primary customers, used "skins" when they had sex with their clients. They also sold condoms for use with other women.

In the 19th century rubber condoms were available, but they were often of poor quality.

Latex condoms and mechanization of production in the 1930s permitted the manufacture of higher quality condoms for sale at affordable prices.

Although "skins" are still available, they are expensive. More than 95% of condoms sold worldwide are now made of latex.

Wide availability of wonder drugs such as penicillin, new contraceptive methods not associated with the sex act such as the "pill," and easier access to abortion brought about the "sexual revolution." The mode of behavior for many men and women was "going natural." Condom use declined.

But the 1980s brought an end to the sexual revolution —and to the declining use of condoms.

New strains of gonorrhea and syphilis resistant to antibiotics emerged. Antibiotics were still as close as the nearest doctor, but they could no longer be relied upon to provide a magic cure for an STD infection.

Moreover, new diseases appeared. Herpes came first. It is not currently curable, but it is not usually fatal.

Next came AIDS which is fatal. A person may be infected with the AIDS virus and be capable of transmitting it to others without the victim displaying outward signs of the disease and without his or her even knowing of the infection.

Condoms provide the only protection against AIDS for people who engage in sexual relations with partners whose infection status is uncertain.

But the condom should not be viewed only as a prophylactic against sexually transmitted diseases. It is also a contraceptive quite appropriate for use within as well as outside marriage. Half of all Japanese couples use the condom as their primary contraceptive method.

#2 Origins of Condoms

Ancient Times

How long have people used condoms?

Ancient Egyptian art dating back more than 3,000 years shows men with sheaths over the glans of their penises.

Were these sheaths ancient condoms intended to provide protection against sexually transmitted disease and pregnancy?

Or jockstraps to protect against physical injury during combat, sports or heavy labor?

Or were they cosmetic? Adornments to beautify the male anatomy?

Or was modesty the motivating factor?

Egyptian literature does not provide an answer to the riddle. An Egyptian papyrus containing recipes for contraceptives exists, but it is badly damaged. Some of the recipes can not be deciphered.

Condoms were not among the prescriptions in the legible portion of the document, so the Egyptian sheaths remain a mystery.

Roman legend refers to the use of a goat's bladder as a type of female condom. The bladder was placed in the vagina to form a pouch to receive the penis and trap semen.

Unlike the Egyptian sheaths, the purpose of the goat's bladder is clear. But it is not clear whether the legend reflects actual practice in Roman society.

Sixteenth To Eighteenth Century Innovations

The 16th century Italian anatomist Fallopius (for whom the tubes through which human eggs transit from the ovaries to the uterus were named) described a linen sheath cut to shape for the glans of the penis. Although his device is an early forerunner of the modern condom, his interest was in preventing syphilis rather than pregnancy.

By the 18th century European workmen engaged in meat processing had a lively business making condoms from animal intestines.

Condoms were in wide use by European prostitutes of the period. They provided a retail outlet for the devices.

The famed lover Casanova was one of many 18th century writers who recorded personal experience with condoms.

About the time of the American Revolution, handbills advertising condoms appeared on the streets of London. Since the messages on the handbills assumed considerable knowledge of condoms, a substantial segment of London society must have known of them.

Development of Rubber and Latex Condoms

Vulcanization of rubber in the 1840s led to the development of rubber condoms later in the 19th century. Rubber condoms cost less than those made of animal skin. Consequently, more people could afford to buy them. However, one source estimated that three quarters of these early rubber condoms were defective.

The development of latex and the mechanization of production in the 1930s permitted the manufacture of high quality condoms at popular prices.

Today, most condoms are made from latex, although some are still made from animal membrane.

The Changing Image of Condoms

Condoms have had a long-term tainted image. Their early association with prostitution follows them to the present day.

In the late 19th century, condoms were condemned by the medical profession as unnatural, immoral and dangerous.

Among other outlets, condoms were also sold in pool rooms, filling stations and barber shops. They were outlawed in many states and were labeled "Sold for the Prevention of Disease Only" in many, adding to the negative image.

In the 1920s Merle Youngs, a salesman of drug products, began making condoms for sale exclusively to drugstores. He also filed lawsuits challenging state laws which banned condom sales.

High quality condoms offering a variety of features are now marketed. The features include:

- Different sizes
- Different shapes
- Different textures
- Various thicknesses
- Several colors
- Various degrees and types of lubrication
- Addition of spermicidal agents

Reference: 12, 21

Notes

#3 Modern Uses for Condoms

Purpose of Condom Use

Condoms are used for two primary purposes:

- Prevention of pregnancy
- Prevention of disease

Condoms can be an effective means of family planning when used properly and regularly. They can also be an effective tool for controlling sexually transmitted diseases (STDs).

Prior to the development of antibiotics, condoms were used extensively to control STDs. However, when penicillin became widely available after the Second World War, people became lax in their behavior. If an infection developed, a shot of penicillin was as close as the nearest doctor.

The arrival of the "Pill" in the 1960s provided a highly effective and easy-to-use means of preventing unwanted pregnancies. "Going natural" felt better than wearing a condom, while penicillin and the Pill removed the fear.

The sexual revolution was in full swing. As a consequence of repeated use of antibiotics, new strains of gonorrhea and other STDs developed that were extremely resistant to ordinary antibiotics. The sexual revolution also saw the spread of herpes, which could be controlled but not cured.

STDs were viewed as little more than unpleasant annoyances. "In Search Of" ads in city magazines readily acknowledged herpes infections and advertised for understanding partners.

Then there was AIDS, the killer disease. At first, the "straight" community shrugged off the growing number of AIDS victims, calling it the "gay plague," but AIDS is now widely acknowledged to be a deadly threat to "gays" and "straights" alike. In fact, AIDS appears to be spreading more slowly among gays and more rapidly among straights.

Condoms provide the only means whereby couples can engage in sexual activity with some degree of protection, although there is increasing concern about how effective condoms are in protecting against AIDS (see Section #11).

Campaigns to Increase Condom Use

The AIDS pandemic spurred campaigns in various countries to encourage condom use. The campaign in Great Britain took a remarkably direct approach. It was largely devoid of moral preaching, concentrating instead on providing straightforward information on safe sex, the threat of AIDS, and the proper use of condoms.

The United States, on the other hand, initially took a more abstract approach with a high degree of preachment and little basic information, reflecting the Reagan administration's negative views on sex, birth control, and homosexuality. The programs were largely ineffective.

A new, much more direct approach emerged. The programs now provide not only basic information on safe sex practices but also free condoms. Some junior and senior high schools distribute or plan to distribute condoms to both boys and girls upon request. It remains to be seen whether the predictable opposition from the Catholic bishops and others who believe that distributing condoms to teenagers only serves to encourage sexual activity will block the programs. The deadly nature of AIDS and the annual one million teenage pregnancies in the United States will no doubt spur many school districts to proceed with their programs despite the opposition.

Levels of Effectiveness

Condoms do not provide 100 percent protection from either pregnancy or STDs. The level of protection they provide is thought to be highly dependent upon user behavior (see Section #9). Twenty-five to thirty percent of couples using condoms carelessly and sporadically experience a resulting pregnancy. Used correctly and regularly, pregnancy rates fall to less than five percent and possibly as low as one or two percent.

Condoms probably offer greater protection against pregnancy than they do against disease. Women are at risk of becoming pregnant only a few days each month. Condom failure during the rest of the month will not result in a pregnancy.

But both partners are at risk of infection for the entire month.

Medical authorities point out that the AIDS virus is fragile and hard to transmit. They also point out that the consequence of contracting AIDS is likely to be death.

Condoms can reduce but not erase the risk of transmitting AIDS. Medical authorities are becoming more realistic about the degree of protection condoms provide — or rather more willing to acknowledge that they really do not know.

Many laboratory experiments have shown that latex is impervious to virus, including AIDS, but very little is known about the effectiveness of latex condoms in actual use (see Section #8).

In a survey of its readers, *Consumer Reports* found that one condom user in four had experienced a break in the past year. Nearly one in eight had two breakages. *Consumer Reports* estimates the breakage rate at one per 140 condoms (Ref 27).

#4 Female-Oriented Contraceptive Methods

Bearers of the Burden

A line from the Broadway musical, "Kiss Me, Kate," sums up the stereotypical roles of men and women in human sexuality and reproduction:

"It's he who'll have the fun and thee the baby."

Although this caricature is an unfair assessment of many men's sense of responsibility, it is true that the burden of pregnancy and family planning falls disproportionately on women.

Most contraceptive methods are female-oriented. A woman may choose any one or sometimes a combination of the available methods, including:

- Oral contraceptives (the "Pill")
- An intrauterine device (IUD)
- A diaphragm
- Vaginal sponges
- Vaginal spermicidal jelly
- Implanted contraceptive capsules
- Contraceptive injections
- Surgical sterilization (generally, a tubectomy or "tying the tubes")

All of these methods require action by the female but not by the male partner.

Periodic abstinence (the "rhythm method") requires action - or non-action - by both partners, who must forego vaginal intercourse during periods deemed to be at highest risk for pregnancy. These determinations may be made by:

- Charting the female partner's usual menstrual cycles (the "calendar" method)
- Careful recording of morning temperature (the "temperature" method) to pinpoint the time of ovulation
- Testing the consistency of the mucus in the vagina to determine the time of ovulation (the "dip stick" or "Billings" method)

Male-oriented methods of contraception are covered in a separate section (see Section #5).

#5 Male-Oriented Contraceptive Methods

The Various Methods

There are four major male-oriented methods of contraception. They are:

- Coitus reservatus
- Coitus interruptus
- Vasectomy
- Condom

Rates of use vary: coitus reservatus is rare, while the other three methods are, in some degree, in common use in one or more parts of the world.

Coitus Reservatus

Coitus reservatus is also called "male continence" because it requires the male to "reserve" or not release his sperm. It has never been a widely popular method of contraception.

The method had its origin in an erroneous understanding of male physiology and specifically in the mistaken belief that, at birth, males had a limited, nonrenewable supply of semen. It was believed that once this supply was used up, sexual activity ended and the aging process accelerated.

By conserving the supply of semen, it was assumed, sex life could be extended and aging delayed.

Practice of the method required the male to put his penis into his partner's vagina with the goal of having an orgasm without ejaculating.

Two approaches to this end are mentioned in the literature:

In one, the male minimizes penis movement, concentrating on the spiritual side of sex (Ref 11).

In the other, the male thrusts until his sexual excitement builds. He then stops thrusting but does not withdraw his penis. As arousal subsides, he may resume thrusting until another urge builds.

The couple may repeat the process for as long as they like (Ref 11).

Current knowledge of the method seems to be quite limited. Surveys of family planning knowledge and use in recent years do not report its use.

It was advocated in 17th century Japan, Victorian England and elsewhere, more for its assumed physiological value than as a method of birth control.

In the United States, a 19th century communal society near Oneida, New York used it as the birth control method of choice. Coitus reservatus may have some appeal as an occasional sexual variation rather than as a regular birth control method, but couples who choose to experiment may wish to use another contraceptive as well to protect against accidental ejaculation or stray sperm.

Coitus Interruptus

Coitus interruptus requires the male to withdraw his penis prior to ejaculation to deposit his semen outside the vagina. The method is ancient and is mentioned in the Bible.

Genesis (38:6-10) provides the following account:

> And Judah took a wife for Er his firstborn, and her name was Tamar.
>
> And Er, Judah's firstborn, was wicked in the sight of the Lord; and the Lord slew him.
>
> Then Judah said to Onan: "Go in to your brother's wife, and perform the duty of a brother-in-law to her, and raise up offspring for your brother."
>
> But Onan knew that the offspring would not be his; so when he went in to his brother's wife, he spilled his semen on the ground, lest he should give offspring to his brother.
>
> And what he did was displeasing in the sight of the Lord; and He slew him also.

The passage has been variously interpreted as condemning coitus interruptus, contraception generally, or masturbation, which also involves "spilling semen on the ground."

Onan engaged in coitus interruptus, not masturbation, but the real issue here was Onan's disobedience of Talmudic law requiring him to impregnate his sister-in-law to continue his dead brother's line.

Under Hebrew inheritance law, property passed to first-born sons. Had Onan sired a son for his older brother, the son rather than Onan would be in line to inherit the family property. Thus, one interpretation is that Onan's sin was greed.

Coitus interruptus played a major role in European fertility declines during the 19th and early

20th centuries. It is still a major birth control method in Europe (Ref 11, 17).

Table 1 shows use rates for countries where 10% or more of couples use coitus interruptus, as determined by surveys carried out in recent years.

Fully 60 percent of Bulgarian couples and 36 percent of Italian and Yugoslavian couples use coitus interruptus. In comparison, only one percent of American couples use this method, according to fertility surveys.

Because coitus interruptus requires quick action by the male, who must withdraw abruptly at the height of sexual excitement, one or both sexual partners may find the practice frustrating.

Vasectomy

Vasectomy (male sterilization) involves cutting or blocking the vas deferens, the tubes that carry sperm from the testes into the pelvic area where they are mixed with other components of semen preparatory to ejaculation.

Worldwide, about 50 million men have elected to have vasectomies. Table 2 lists four countries where five percent or more of reproductive age couples rely on vasectomy as their family planning method of choice.

Vasectomy is often performed in the doctor's office with a local anesthesia. The patient sometimes has the option of watching the procedure in an overhead mirror.

The wife may also have the option of being present during the operation. Just as some couples choose to share the experience of the birth of their children, some also may elect to be together during the vasectomy procedure which marks an end to their childbearing years.

Although surgery of any kind carries some risk, serious complications of vasectomy are rare. The procedure may cause some men to experience a few days of discomfort, but many are able to return to work the next day.

Contraceptive effectiveness of a vasectomy is not immediate. It takes a few weeks for the sperm in the male reproductive tract to be cleared out. Another method of contraception should be used during that period.

Vasectomy does not affect sexual function. Sperm make up only two percent of semen. Most of the components of semen are produced by a series of glands in the pelvic area, so vasectomized men rarely observe a difference in the quantity of semen they ejaculate.

Vasectomy is an effective and appropriate way for men to take responsibility for family planning when a couple has had all the children they want.

Notes

#6 International Condom Use

Growing Numbers of Users Worldwide

At least 50 million couples use condoms, and the number appears to be growing, sparked by the spread of AIDS and knowledge that condoms offer the only protection against the disease except sexual abstinence.

The data on condom use in Table 3 are from surveys taken before the impact of the AIDS pandemic on condom use.

Japan: World's Largest Condom User

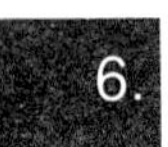

Half of all Japanese couples rely on condoms as their primary contraceptive method. In terms of numbers, the Japanese use about one-quarter of worldwide condom production. Condoms are marketed in Japan through a network of saleswomen who go door-to-door selling mainly to housewives.

The primary reason for Japanese reliance on condoms is the limited contraceptive choices available to them. The Japanese Government has not approved the Pill for use as a general contraceptive, and most other methods are not popular for a variety of cultural reasons.

During the American occupation after World War II, abortion came into wide use as a means of family planning for individual couples and to limit Japan's population to the number the Home Islands could support. Condoms were later promoted as a means of reducing the high abortion rate.

Japanese couples now use condoms in conjunction with abortion for family planning.

Condom Use Elsewhere

At the time the surveys were taken (mostly prior to 1984), several European countries had fairly high condom use rates. One-third of couples in Finland and one-fourth of those in Denmark use condoms.

In the Third World, 17 percent of couples in Trinidad and Tobago and 12 percent of those in Taiwan use condoms.

Five years ago when the survey of contraceptive use in the United States was taken, about 10 percent of American couples used condoms.

Public statements by executives of American condom companies indicate that the number of American couples using condoms has doubled since 1982.

The next round of contraceptive prevalence surveys is expected to show dramatically higher use rates for condoms, but the results of the surveys will not be available until the early 1990's.

Evidence of Rising Condom Use

Requests for condoms to the US International Population Program have been rising rapidly, particularly for areas of the world such as Africa, where AIDS is widespread.

According to an article in *Playboy*, the United States Agency for International Development (USAID) - not to be confused with AIDS (acquired immunodeficiency syndrome) - provided 234 million condoms to Third World nations in 1981, an increase of almost 100 million from the previous year. By 1984, the number reached 560 million and, in 1985, 568 million (Ref 5).

Through 1985, few USAID condoms were shipped to Africa, but the AIDS pandemic coupled with an increasing interest in family planning caused condom shipments to skyrocket. USAID shipments of condoms to eight African countries between 1984 and September 1989 are given in Table 8.

In 1984, nearly 5.4 million condoms were shipped to these eight countries. In 1985, the number tripled to 15.4 million. By 1988, some 46 million condoms, nine times as many as in 1984, were sent; and, in the first nine months of 1989, the number reached nearly 39.5 million (Ref 28).

Notes

#7 Agreeing on Condom Use

Raising the Subject

Many people say that insisting on condom use is awkward, and that the task falls heaviest on the partner who first brings up the subject.

The reasons for condom use are obvious. If used correctly, condoms are not only a safe and effective method of birth control, they are the only currently available method for people who are sexually active with partners whose infection status is not known to reduce the risk of spreading sexually transmitted diseases, including AIDS.

So why do people get upset about asking their partner to use a condom?

The major difficulty, when a person feels awkward introducing the subject, is that they are often concerned that they will sound as if they are accusing their partner (of being diseased, untrustworthy, "gay", etc.).

First, the subject should be discussed in a comfortable time and place, not at the moment of passion.

Second, the best way to avoid the problem of sounding accusatory is to use an approach which:

- Voices personal concerns
- Is non-threatening or non-accusatory
- Is reassuring to the other partner

Use of a personal focus helps to diminish the awkwardness for the other partner. For example, ways to bring up the subject in a non-threatening manner include:

- "I've been seeing a lot of ads lately on TV (or in the magazines, in the newspapers, in the stores) about condoms, and it started me thinking..."
- "I really feel uncomfortable mentioning this, but I've been thinking... "
- "Just recently, I was talking to a person I know, and she (he) and her (his) husband (wife, friend, lover) are using condoms now. It really started me thinking..."
- "I've been really frightened by what I'm hearing about diseases like AIDS spreading and people not even knowing they'd been exposed. I can't stop feeling afraid, but I was thinking..."
- We've both been so conscious of trying to protect our health (diet, exercise, etc.), it seems like another way to protect ourselves might be ...."

These are just a few suggestions, but they all share an approach to the topic that focuses on the feelings of the partner who has introduced the subject, and does not directly accuse or attack the other partner. This approach can be adapted to most situations, whether the relationship is of short or long duration.

Assertion

Discussion of the subject, as outlined above, is an approach particularly suited to those who wish to reassure their partners. The longer the relationship, the more necessary the reassuring introduction of the subject.

Some individuals, especially those whose sexual relationship is just beginning or has been of relatively short duration, can simply skip the discussion and begin with the assertion that they expect their partner to use condoms. Some women may avoid awkwardness by providing condoms to their partners.

The assertion can be handled in the same personal, non-threatening manner as the discussion. For example:

- "I think we ought to use condoms."
- "It only makes sense to use condoms."
- "I think we need to protect each other and use condoms."
- "We have so much to lose. Let's be safe."
- "It's really worth it to be safe, and use condoms."

These suggestions can be modified to fit the situation.

Another approach is to be direct and matter of fact. In one television spot, the couple (who presumably are about to have sex for the first time) are shown in the woman's bedroom. As she enters the bathroom, she tells her partner, "The condoms are in the table by the bed."

Resistance

When one partner brings up the subject of condom use, makes the statement that they want to use condoms, and the other partner accepts it, then there will probably be no further difficulty.

However, sometimes the situation is not so simple. The other partner may not agree to use condoms or may not agree initially. In this circumstance, the partner who has suggested condom use should not give up, but should let the non-accepting partner voice his (or her) concerns, and should respond to those concerns in as positive and reassuring a manner as possible.

Some men, and less often women, resist condom use, citing reasons which include:

- Insulted feelings
- Rejection of condoms themselves
  - Condoms feel different
  - Condoms look different
- Interruption of sexual mood with condom use
- Past difficulty in using condoms
- Rejection of "image" of condoms
- Assertion that condoms are not effective
- Denial of danger requiring condom use

A man rejecting condom use on the basis of being insulted has often taken the suggestion as a personal attack. He may say that he is being accused of being untrustworthy, diseased, etc. One approach is to return to the discussion of the subject and begin again, reassuring him. Example: "I know it seems like it questions the trust between us, but there is a serious national health problem with AIDS and other sexually transmitted diseases. One of the difficulties is that a person can be exposed to some of these diseases and not even realize it. It's because I want us to take care of ourselves and to protect one another that I'm suggesting we use condoms."

Rejection of condoms themselves, the complaint that they disturb the mood of passion and the argument that past use of condoms has been unsatisfactory are all based on lack of practice with condoms. All can be handled with gentle reassurance and the partner's willingness to help: "I know it may take some getting used to, but I really think it's important that we use condoms. Let's make it a project: we can try as many brands as you like to find one that you feel comfortable with ."

Arguments about effectiveness have some degree of validity: condoms are not 100% effective. Nothing is. But even the Surgeon General of the United States has said that condoms are the only method available for sexually active people to protect themselves against the AIDS virus. Condoms plus spermicide offer the best protection possible.

Denial of the possibility of danger which would require use of condoms can take several forms. Often, the denial is based on misinformation. The rejecting partner may insist that he or she simply does not have a disease nor have they been exposed to a disease. The problem is that few sexually active people can make a declaration with complete, 100% assurance that they have had no sex partner from the past ten years who was ever exposed to the virus or that the disease might not have been transmitted to them or a sex partner through a transfusion or other method. The response might be: "I know it doesn't seem like it could happen, but the risks are so great if we're mistaken, and taking precautions is so easy. I'd feel so much better just to know that I'd done all I could to protect you and protect myself."

The most important point, in countering resistance, is to try to understand the objections and feelings of the other partner and to offer reassurance while continuing to insist, gently but firmly, on use of condoms.

Insistence

If discussion fails, some partners are forced to insist that condoms be used or else no sexual activity which involves exchange of body fluids will take place.

Activities that medical authorities consider to be safe without condom use include:

- Hugging
- Dry kissing
- Massaging

Other activities, such as mutual masturbation, carry more risk, particularly if care is not taken to avoid the exchange of body fluids. But medical authorities consider these practices safer than sexual activities that involve penetration.

Open sores and cuts provide a potential avenue of entry for HIV infection and should be viewed with concern. They may be reason enough to avoid sexual activity.

#8 Measuring Effectiveness

Kinds of Effectiveness Rates

Scientists concerned with contraceptive effectiveness employ two concepts: "theoretical effectiveness" and "use effectiveness."

"Theoretical effectiveness" reflects laboratory or ideal conditions where many factors influencing effectiveness can be controlled. "Use effectiveness" reflects what actually happens when the contraceptive is used by ordinary people under ordinary conditions.

The effectiveness of a contraceptive is expressed in terms of the number of pregnancies occurring to 100 couples who use the method for a year.

If the 100 couples have five pregnancies, the failure rate is five, or five percent.

Another way of conveying the same information is to emphasize that 95 of the 100 couples did not experience a pregnancy. Thus, the effectiveness rate for the method is 95, or 95 percent.

To make the information more meaningful to individual couples, the failure rate may also be expressed in terms of the average number of unplanned pregnancies a couple might experience if they used the method for their entire reproductive lifetime without stopping to have a planned birth.

Twenty-five years is the approximate reproductive period for a typical couple who marry at about age 23 and remain married until the woman reaches menopause in her late forties. Thus, the experience of 100 couples for a year is approximately equal to the lifetime experience of four couples.

A contraceptive method with a failure rate of 4 means that couples using the method throughout their reproductive lifetime will average one unplanned pregnancy. A failure rate of 8 means an average of two unplanned pregnancies per couple.

Note that these are statistical averages. The experiences of individual couples are influenced by a wide range of factors and may be different from the average.

Use Effectiveness Rates for Condoms

Used properly, condoms can be highly effective. Pregnancy rates around one percent are probably attainable if a spermicide is used along with the condom, and proper condom use procedures are followed (see Sections #13 and #14).

Regrettably, many people use condoms sporadically and improperly. Under these circumstances, failure rates can reach 20 or more. Not only does this represent unwanted pregnancies, it means that the condom user is also failing to achieve any real degree of protection from sexually transmitted diseases.

At this level of effectiveness (or ineffectiveness), couples would average five unplanned pregnancies during their reproductive lifetimes.

The highest failure rates are found among young people who lack basic knowledge of sexuality, reproduction and contraception.

#9 Behavior Affecting Condom Use

Factors in Effectiveness

Factors with an impact on the condom's effectiveness in preventing pregnancy and disease are:

- Motivation
- Sexual behavior
- Proper use of the condom (see Sections #13 and #14)

Motivation

The motivation to prevent disease or pregnancy can be overwhelmed in a moment of passion. The sex drive, particularly among young people, is extremely powerful. It can overpower cultural and religious prohibitions as well as fears of pregnancy and disease, including the killer disease AIDS, even among people who under other circumstances are quite responsible.

Experience since the AIDS pandemic began indicates that information programs may teach people what constitutes appropriate behavior, but that knowledge does not necessarily lead to behavior modification.

One study among male homosexuals in San Francisco found that while 80 percent said they were aware of the recommendation to use condoms to reduce AIDS transmission, fewer than five percent were doing so (Ref 24).

A spokesmen for the San Francisco gay community asserted that the study was dated because it was carried out before the gay community had completed the transition in sexual behavior that took place in that community.

The spread of AIDS among gay men in areas like San Francisco and New York may be abating. Health authorities do not agree on the reasons, however.

Among gay and bisexual men in a study population in San Francisco, the annual AIDS infection rate increased as follows:

- 22.8% in the last half of 1982
- 48.6% in the last half of 1984
- 50% thereafter

The percentage of increase in the annual infection rates in this population began to decline during this same period (Ref 25) as follows:

- 18.4% increase per year from 1982 to 1984
- 8.5% increase during 1985 (5.4% during 1st half; 3.1% during 2nd half of year)
- 4.2% increase for 1st half of 1986

Some credit powerful information programs for behavior modification. Others attribute the slowdown to a dwindling supply of susceptible people in this particular community.

Sexual Behavior

The more sexual partners a person has, the more he or she is at risk. AIDS is a particularly dangerous disease because it is possible for a person to be infected and carry the virus for years (some experts say up to 10) without developing any outward signs. It is probable that the person would not even know he/she had been infected. Yet he or she would still be contagious and capable of infecting others.

Moreover, some reports are appearing that even people who know they are infected with the virus may not tell others, including people with whom they have sex. Motives for people behaving in this irresponsible manner include:

- Fear of rejection
- Anger at their own (terminal) illness
- Revenge on those as yet uninfected
- Fear of lost income

Avenues of Transmission

AIDS may be transmitted by all forms of sexual intercourse - vaginal, anal, and oral.

AIDS may also be transmitted through a variety of non-sexual means to individuals in a previously uninfected population and then spread both sexually and non-sexually through the new group. For this reason, people should screen prospective sex partners for potential exposure to AIDS through both sexual and non-sexual means.

Medical authorities have been quick to reassure the public that AIDS cannot be passed through this or that mechanism. The reassurances often have taken the form of such statements as "There is no *known* case of AIDS being transmitted by ...."Authorities claimed, for example, that women could not transmit AIDS to male sex partners, but women *have* infected male partners.

Authorities also claimed that AIDS-infected health providers did not pose a threat to their patients, but it is now acknowledged that AIDS was transmitted from at least one dentist to several of his patients. The dentist and at least one of his patients died of the disease.

Currently, the blood supply is said to be safe, but some people who were infected earlier from blood transfusions or the use of drugs made from blood products may develop the disease at a future time. Moreover, there is still a possibility that HIV-infected blood may get through the screening process.

IV drug users can and do contract AIDs through the use of dirty needles, and drug addicts sometimes exchange sex for drugs or sell sex in order to obtain money to buy drugs.

Since licensed medical facilities in most developed countries use presterilized needles that are discarded after use, patients receiving injections have virtually no risk of catching AIDS from injections. However, medical personnel have been infected when they were accidentally pricked by a used needle. Theoretically, patients could also be pricked by a contaminated needle left over from another patient, but the chances are probably quite small.

Medical units in developing countries often re-use needles. The sterilization process may not kill all the microorganisms, so contaminated needles in legitimate medical units may be one of the avenues for AIDS transmission in developing countries.

People have contracted AIDS from blood transfusions and from infusion of blood products or derivatives.

Hemophiliacs receive injections of a blood derivative containing the clotting factor of other people's blood. Some hemophiliacs have contracted AIDS from these injections.

Blood products may contain antibodies to the AIDS virus but no live virus. Since the most common test for AIDS checks for the existence of antibodies, people receiving injections of these products may test positive for AIDS but not have the disease.

Insects are known carriers of diseases like yellow fever and malaria. Insects bite to obtain blood from their victims. When they bite a person with malaria, for example, the blood they obtain may contain the organisms that cause malaria. When they bite a second person, some of the blood from the first is injected into the blood stream of the second.

Most public health professionals assert that there are no known cases of AIDS transmission by insect bites. They point to the fact that in Africa, where AIDS is widespread, children between ages 2 and 13 rarely contract it. Insects bite everyone, so if AIDS were being transmitted by insects, African children should be getting it in larger numbers.

Other possible avenues of transmission include tattooing and ear-piercing outside medical facilities.

Following the overthrow of the Romanian dictator Nicolae Ceausescu in December 1989, large numbers of children with AIDS were discovered in government institutions. These children probably contracted AIDS from the practice of a weird medical procedure apparently ordered by the medically-illiterate dictator and his wife. The children were given periodic injections of blood for some supposed medical benefit. The blood used in this quackery was largely collected at the Black Sea port of Constanta where AIDS seemed to be widespread among seamen and dock workers.

This avenue of AIDS transmission was totally unexpected by the international AIDS experts. The warehouses of surplus children in Romania resulted from Ceausescu's outlawing of both abortion and contraceptives.

When It Is Safe Not to Use Condoms

There has been much recent debate among medical experts about the Issue of when sex is safe, in terms of exposure to sexually transmitted diseases. Another version of this question is: when is it safe not to use a condom?

There are two situations where the answer to the question is clear:

- Condoms are mandatory when an individual has many sex partners or engages in sex in high-risk situations (such as with prostitutes or at sex clubs)
- Condoms are not required when a couple has maintained a faithful monogamous relationship for a long time

The dilemma is that the greater majority of sexually-active people fall between these two extremes.

Prudence dictates that condoms be used in new relationships. However, in continuing long-term relationships, the question of safety depends primarily on whether the relationship is mutually monogamous.

Couples often have difficulty being either totally faithful or totally honest about behavior that could put the other partner at risk.

Some medical authorities recommend that, for a high degree of safety, a couple planning to establish a safely monogamous relationship follow these procedures:

- Do not engage in intercourse until cleared of sexually- transmitted diseases (especially AIDS)
- Undergo an AIDS screening
- If the test is clear, wait six months — during which time no sexual practices involving an exchange of body fluids should take place between the partners or between either partner and anyone else
- Undergo another AIDS screening
- If the second test is clear, the partners are probably safe to begin a sexual relationship — as long as they remain strictly monogamous (Ref 18)

These rules assume both partners are not using intravenous drugs. They also assume that the partners have considered other avenues of possible AIDS transmission such as those discussed above.

These recommendations sound very harsh, but the medical professionals who list them emphasize that this is the only currently available answer to the question of safety.

NOTES

#10 Safer Sex

What constitutes safe sex?

The safest sex is solitary masturbation. Studies of sexual behavior indicate that virtually all males and a large majority of females masturbate at some stage in their lives. The AIDS pandemic may well add to the popularity of the practice.

Since most people prefer sex with someone else, the safest sex with a partner involves avoidance of penetration and other behavior leading to an exchange of body fluids.

When penetration does occur, condoms provide the only currently available protection.

The More Partners, the Greater the Risk

Public health officials emphasize that the risk of contracting AIDS grows as the number of sexual partners rises.

They warn that, with respect to AIDS, a person having sex is, in practical terms, having sex with all the people their partner has had sex with and all of the people those people have had sex with, for the past 7 to 10 years.

Numbers can build rapidly, as demonstrated by the figures in Table 5. The first column of numbers shows what would happen if an individual had two new sex partners each year, each of whom also had two new partners. Just two new sex partners per year for seven years means direct exposure to 14 partners and indirect exposure to 490 additional partners for a total exposure to 504 people.

The second column shows what would happen if each person had three new partners each year. Three partners annually means direct and indirect exposure to 4,905 people during a seven year period.

How Effective is the Condom in Preventing AIDS?

Medical authorities talk about condom use as the only means, short of sexual abstinence, of avoiding AIDS.

But how effective is the condom in preventing transmission of AIDS?

There are numerous reports in the medical literature about laboratory experiments whereby condoms are subjected to forces similar to those encountered during sexual intercourse to determine how effective condoms are in containing viruses, including the AIDS virus. But relatively little is known about the effectiveness of condoms in actual use by human beings.

Among the items cited in Section #9 are field studies of AIDS transmission among prostitutes, but how relevant these studies are outside the commercial sex market is not known.

Medical authorities are beginning to face up to this sad fact of life and death in this terrifying age. New research to answer some of the questions will likely be initiated in the near future, but the results may not be available for months or years.

Since few people will wish to practice abstinence over an extended period of their lives, condoms do offer substantial protection, particularly if used regularly and correctly.

Ignoring the Risk

Until recently, there has been a tendency among some people to rationalize failure to follow safe sex prescriptions by asserting that AIDS is a disease which only affects gays and intravenous drug-users.

It is because of such short-sighted and ill-informed rationalizations that many choose not to protect themselves or their sexual partners against the disease, secure in the mistaken belief that it could not strike them.

However, in Africa, AIDS is primarily found among heterosexuals. The male-to-female infection rate is about one to one, versus a ratio to date of nine males to one female in the United States. The African data clearly demonstrates that the disease is capable of being spread in both directions between men and women, and it could happen in the United States.

Currently, in the United States, the number of gay men afflicted by the disease seems to be decreasing while incidence is increasing among heterosexuals who do not belong to any of the groups previously thought to be at high risk. One common denominator, though, may be the rationalization that it could not happen to them.

Condom Use and Disease Transmission

Recommended procedures governing condom use for disease prevention are very different from those relating to pregnancy prevention. Even brief unprotected genital contact poses a risk of disease transmission. Using condoms as casually as many couples have used them in the past is an open invitation to infection by sexually transmitted diseases, including AIDS.

Condoms can and do break. Most breaks are probably associated with improper use, but there is an undetermined risk of breakage in normal use.

Consumer Reports surveyed its readers about their experience with condoms. One in four condom users reported that they had experienced condom breakage during the past year and nearly one in eight reported two breaks. Using these data and reports on the number of condoms used, *Consumer Reports* estimates that one condom in 140 breaks.

The breakage rate was much higher for condoms used in anal intercourse (one in 105) than those used in vaginal intercourse (one in 165). Anal intercourse is not exclusively male to male. Ten percent of heterosexual males surveyed by *Consumer Reports* said they had engaged in male to female anal intercourse using a condom (Ref 27).

When breaks do occur, prompt use of a spermicide may reduce the risk of disease transmission as well as the risk of pregnancy.

The spermicide Nonoxynol-9 does kill the AIDS virus in laboratory experiments, but its effectiveness in actual use remains to be established.

Body fluids can seep into or out of condoms around the rim. This risk can be reduced by the following procedures:

- The condom should have a reservoir tip to trap semen
- The penis should be entirely covered by the condom

- The penis should be withdrawn while it is still erect
- The rim of the condom should be held to prevent spillage while withdrawing

Body fluids may be spread to the hands and other body parts. Careful washing of hands and areas contacted can also reduce the risk of disease transmission.

Anal Intercourse

Anal intercourse is unsafe and can be extremely dangerous. It is particularly unsafe for the passive or receptive partner in both homosexual and heterosexual relationships (Ref 6). The intestine is much more susceptible than the vagina to:

- Trauma
- Tearing of tissues
- Bleeding
- Infection

Those who insist on engaging in this practice regardless of the risk are better protected from disease transmission when using a condom, but they should be aware that the risk of condom breakage is substantially higher for anal intercourse than for vaginal intercourse.

Misinformation

A surprisingly large number of people, particularly the young, have limited or erroneous knowledge of reproductive physiology which affects their contraceptive behavior.

For example, some people believe that pregnancy can occur only when both partners climax at the same time.

This myth may have originated in a mistaken understanding of reproductive physiology dating back at least to Greek and Roman times.

Prior to the invention of the microscope in the 17th century, people had no knowledge of micro-organisms, including sperm and ova. Semen was believed to contain the complete seed of life. It was thought that a woman contributed nothing to the genetics of the fetus in her womb and that her role was limited to providing the "soil" into which the man could "plant his seed." Since men were seen to "plant their seed" many times when only a few sprouted, the ancients believed that something in the female must control whether the seed reached fertile soil or fell on barren ground.

Since it could be observed that the male climax resulted in the ejaculation of semen, a seeming logical parallel was a belief that the female climax was associated with the opening of the womb to admit semen.

However, we now know that timing of climax has no effect whatsoever on impregnation. Motile sperm deposited in the vagina will endeavor to travel up the birth canal in search of an egg to impregnate, and a woman can become pregnant regardless of whether or not she has experienced a climax.

#11 Disease Prevention

Overview

Since protection against sexually-transmitted diseases is an important reason why condom use is increasing, scientists perform tests to determine their effectiveness with respect to specific diseases.

Specific viruses tested include those responsible for:

- Hepatitis B
- Cytomegalovirus
- Herpes simplex
- AIDS

To date, laboratory studies indicate that latex (but not animal membrane) condoms are impervious to viruses and that latex condoms withstand the rigors of simulated intercourse in laboratory settings.

These findings are not wholly unexpected. One of the routine quality control procedures performed by latex condom makers is to inflate random condom samples with either air or water to several times their unstretched size, inspecting them for leaks. Water and air molecules are considerably smaller than viruses associated with sexually transmitted diseases. If air and water molecules cannot pass through latex, it is a reasonable assumption that the viruses cannot pass through either.

Laboratory studies also indicate that spermicides are effective in killing viruses. A reasonable

11.

deduction is that latex condoms with spermicide are more effective in preventing disease transmission than condoms alone.

Some of the studies used special populations (i.e., prostitutes) to gain insights on how well condoms perform in ordinary use. How relevant these studies are to people outside these special populations has not been established.

Increasingly, medical authorities are acknowledging the state of ignorance in this area and calling for more research, but it is likely to be months if not years before findings of new research initiatives become available.

Meanwhile, couples not involved in long-standing, faithfully monogamous relationships should follow the "safer sex" rules presented in Section #10.

Hepatitis B Virus

In one test, a mixture containing radioactively-labeled hepatitis B virus was placed in the tips of six commercially available condoms. The condoms were then exposed to mechanically produced vibrations to simulate the rigors of sexual intercourse.

Five latex brands prevented leakage. A sixth brand, made of sheep intestinal membrane, progressively leaked (Ref 15).

Cytomegalovirus

Latex condoms' ability to prevent transmission of cytomegalovirus was tested by a method similar to that used for hepatitis B.

Condoms containing cytomegalovirus were subjected to stretching and trauma similar to that associated with sexual intercourse. The researchers concluded that condoms would minimize transmission of cytomegalovirus via semen in both heterosexual and homosexual intercourse (Ref 13).

Herpes Simplex Virus

In one study, a high concentration of herpes simplex virus (HSV-2) left in contact with a condom for eight hours did not cross the latex barrier (Ref 2).

In another study, sections of stretched condom latex were examined under an electronic microscope. Although the microscope revealed numerous irregularities in the latex, it did not reveal any pores or imperfections that might affect the integrity of the latex. It was concluded that the herpes virus would not be able to penetrate or pass through this barrier (Ref 14).

AIDS

The efficacy of condoms in preventing pass-through of retroviruses was examined. Both AIDS-associated retrovirus (ARV-2) and a mouse retrovirus were used. Latex condoms were found to be impervious to these particular retroviruses (Ref 1).

Another study assessed the effectiveness of condoms in preventing AIDS transmission among prostitutes in Germany.

Only one percent of licensed prostitutes tested positive for AIDS antibodies compared with 20 percent of unlicensed prostitutes. Unlicensed prostitutes are more likely to be intravenous drug users than licensed prostitutes, but the researchers did not believe drug use alone explained the difference.

A study of 448 licensed female prostitutes in Nuernberg found high condom use levels and no HIV (human immunovirus, the AIDS virus) antibodies. Condom use rates for various sexual activities provided by the prostitutes were:

- 80% of those who masturbated clients
- 90% of those who provided oral sex
- 97.5% of those who engaged in vaginal intercourse

Only five percent of the women reported that they allowed anal intercourse. Of these, 55.5% required condom use.

Another study involving prostitutes compared AIDS transmission among heterosexuals in New York and Kingali, Rwanda in central Africa.

In the United States and other developed countries, AIDS spread first among homosexuals. The male to female ratio is approximately 9:1. In Africa, where the disease has spread primarily among heterosexuals, the male to female ratio is approximately 1:1.

Heterosexual transmission of AIDS in Africa was associated in part with prostitutes, who rarely supply or require use of condoms by their customers. In New York, prostitutes began regular use of condoms before the AIDS epidemic. Among those who are not also intravenous drug-users, lower-than-expected rates of infection seem to suggest that condom use may be providing some protective effect against AIDS transmission (Ref 7).

#12 Teaching Condom Use

The Broomstick

Instructions on how and when to use condoms follow in Sections #13 and #14.

Teaching condom use has proven to be a little more difficult task than it might first appear, particularly in Third World countries where literacy levels are low and where many people have limited knowledge of contraception.

Instructions that seem crystal clear to family planning specialists may not be at all clear to others.

A story about instructing Third World men to use condoms may serve as illustration.

A family planning worker went to a village where contraceptives were being introduced for the first time. He called together the men in the village for a presentation on condom use.

At the end of the meeting, he asked whether the men understood how to use condoms. A sea of nodding heads led the worker to conclude that his efforts had succeeded. He left an ample supply of condoms and returned to his office in the city. Some months later, he returned to the village to see how things had gone.

He was shocked to see that most of the women were pregnant. He called a meeting of the men to find out what went wrong.

"Didn't you understand how to use the condom?" he asked.

"Why, yes," one man replied. "Every time we had sex we unrolled a condom on the broomstick - just like you taught us!"

Proud Pete

Other approaches that have been used to teach people how to use condoms include an animated cartoon-book character called "Proud Pete."

"Pete" was developed by the Swedes for use in Third World countries where literacy levels are low.

By rapidly flipping the pages of the cartoon-book, an impression of animation is created. The cartoon shows a relaxed penis rising to attention, then using its arms (a bit of artistic licence) to pull a condom over its head and down its shaft.

The instructions seem clear. Hopefully, people can make the connection between the actions shown by "Pete" and unrolling a real condom on a real penis.

Pictures

Explicit pictures and drawings may be the best way to teach proper condom use. Several organizations have published pamphlets or booklets that leave little room for interpretation.

A pamphlet published by Planned Parenthood in the United States contains a series of drawings of a man in various stages of putting on a condom on his erect penis.

Another pamphlet entitled "EL COND♡M" published in Spanish by Fundacion Mexicana Para Planeacion Familiar AC in Juarez, Mexico, uses a series of cartoon type drawings to get the message across. One frame shows a man pulling a condom over his penis as his partner hugs him from behind. The next two frames show the couple engaging in intercourse, and another shows the woman using an applicator to inject spermicide into her vagina. There is a text to explain the action and to provide additional information, but the pictures are quite clear.

#13 When to Use a Condom

For Protection Against Disease

The best time to put on a condom is as soon as the penis becomes erect and before any direct genital contact.

Putting on a condom can be an enjoyable part of foreplay for both partners.

When the condom is being used to protect against sexually transmitted disease (STD), it must be put on before genital contact. Even brief unprotected contact is risky.

Even in the days when STDs meant diseases like syphilis and gonorrhea, this was good advice. At least these diseases are amenable to treatment with antibiotics (although some strains have lately become resistant). It is also good advice in protection against herpes, which is not currently curable, but whose outbreaks can be controlled.

AIDS, however, has made the consequences of inadequate protection deadly serious. The user must:

- Put on a condom before any genital contact whatsoever
- Dispose of the condom promptly and properly after use, preferably by flushing it down the toilet
- Promptly clean the hands or any other body parts that may have come in contact with body fluids

For Contraceptive Purposes

When condoms are used solely as contraceptives, it is still advisable to put the condom on before beginning intercourse.

Some couples say they prefer not to use a condom until the man is ready to ejaculate. He then withdraws to put on the condom before reentering his partner. In effect, the couple is combining two methods, coitus interruptus and condom use (see Section #5). This practice is risky, although probably less risky that coitus interruptus used alone. If the man fails to withdraw in time, he may impregnate his partner.

Pre-ejaculant fluid may also contain stray sperm, although medical authorities seem to be divided on this issue. Some studies did not find motile sperm in pre-ejaculant fluid if the man had urinated since his last ejaculation.

#14 How to Use a Condom

Steps in Proper Condom Use

The following procedures should be used in putting on a latex condom:

- Remove the condom from the foil or plastic packet (see Section #18)
- Make sure the roll of latex fabric is on the outside of the condom (see Figure 3)
- Remove air from the tip (if the condom has one)
- If the condom does not have a tip, leave a half-inch of latex material at the end of the penis as a reservoir for semen
- Roll the condom down the penis shaft, making sure there are no air pockets

The entire penis should be covered.

The same general procedures are followed with "skins," except that they do not cling to the penis as rubber condoms do. Instead, to compensate for the loose fit, "skins" have elastic bands around the rim to hold the condom on and prevent leakage.

Some condoms have outer packages which are hard to open. Couples in the throes of passion may not have the patience to open the more difficult containers. Capsules for some "skins" were the most difficult to open. Condom users may wish to remove the outer package before the need for a condom arises or practice opening the outer wrapping so that they develop proficiency at removing it.

Lubricants

Petroleum-based lubricants (like vaseline) should not be used in conjunction with condoms because they may weaken the condom fabric.

Non oil-based "personal" lubricants like Today™ and K-YJelly™ may be used. There are also combinations of spermicide and lubricant which provide both lubrication and increased protection against pregnancy and sexually-transmitted disease.

These substances should be put in the vagina rather than on the condom. They should never be put on the penis under the condom because they might cause the condom to slip off or prevent it from clinging to the penis, increasing the risk of seepage of body fluids.

When selecting a lubricant or a lubricant-spermicide combination, read the label carefully to ensure selection of the desired product. Not all lubricants contain spermicides.

Saliva should not be used as a lubricant. It is a poor lubricant, and it is a body fluid which may contain microorganisms. The AIDS virus has been found in saliva. While public health authorities maintain that there is no known case of AIDS transmission through saliva, the possibility does exist.

Personal lubricants are available in drugstores and are made under germ-free conditions.

Removing a Condom

After ejaculation, the condom user should follow these procedures:

- Withdraw the penis while it is still erect

- Hold the condom at its rim (open end) while withdrawing in order to prevent spillage
- Examine the condom for holes as soon as it is taken off the penis. If holes are present, promptly use a spermicide in the vagina
- Dispose of the condom in a way that prevents others from being exposed to its contents. Wrap it in paper tissue or toilet paper before putting it into the trash or flushing it down the toilet
- Urinate to remove residual sperm from the system
- Wash the hands and pubic area to reduce the possibility of transferring body fluids

If protection against sexually transmitted disease is desired, care must be taken to prevent exchange of body fluids in either direction.

The Next Time

Latex condoms should never be reused.

If the couple wishes to have intercourse more than once during a love-making session, a new condom must be used each time.

Continued intercourse after ejaculation with the old condom may force semen down the shaft of the penis where it can seep out into the vagina.

If possible, the man should urinate to remove residual sperm and wash his hands and penis area immediately after each ejaculation.

"Skin" condoms supposedly can be washed and reused. However, laboratory tests have demonstrated that "skins" are less reliable than latex condoms as barriers to viruses.

When "skins" were subjected to the rigors of simulated intercourse, they progressively leaked (see Section #8). In light of these results, "skins" cannot be recommended if the primary reason for using them is protection against disease transmission.

These findings are disquieting. If "skins" do not provide acceptable protection against disease transmission, they may not be any more effective in preventing pregnancy.

#15 Composition

Shapes

A condom sealed in its foil pack is a flat, circular shape. When the foil is broken open, the condom is revealed with the edges rolled up and, usually, a nipple-like tip in the center.

The tip is sometimes called a reservoir or an end (the advertising literature uses several terms). Its purpose is to provide space to capture and hold ejaculated semen.

Unless some provision is made for this fluid, it may be forced between the shaft of the penis and the condom to the rim, where it can leak into the vagina. Most modern condoms come with tips.

If a condom does not have a tip, the user should leave a half-inch of loose condom material at the head of the penis in order to trap ejaculate fluid.

When unrolled onto the penis, the roll should always be on the outside. Thus positioned, the condom unrolls naturally down the shaft of the penis.

Condoms may be straight in shape (like fingers in a glove) or contoured (e.g., shaped like a penis with a wide head and a narrower neck) (see Figure 3). The condom companies promote contoured condoms as being more sensuous.

See Section #16 for classifications by shape and illustrations in Figure 1.

Texture

Condoms may be either smooth or textured.

Two types of texturing are used: rings of raised latex around the shaft of the condom and tiny specks of raised latex on the surface. Some condoms feature both (see Section #16).

Textured condoms are promoted as increasing pleasure for women or for both partners, but an informal survey by *Men's Health* found that most couples could not sense a difference between smooth and textured condoms.

Consumer Reports found that "textured (ribbed) condoms . . . got a mixed reaction from women. A little more than one fourth preferred the texture but nearly an equal number said they would not use such condoms" (Ref 27).

Lubrication

Condoms may be lubricated or dry. Two types of lubricants are used, a "wet" non-oil based substance and a "dry" silicone lubricant.

Although the terms sound similar, there is a difference between a dry condom and a condom lubricated with dry silicone. A dry condom does not have any lubrication, while "dry" silicone lubricant is a fine, slightly damp dust.

Whether to buy lubricated or dry condoms is partly a matter of personal preference, although budget may also be a consideration since dry condoms are sometimes, but not always, cheaper (see Section #19).

Since the primary reason for using condoms is to prevent transfer of body fluids, the normal mixing of lubricating fluids from the two partners is absent.

Comfortable entry of a penis covered by a nonlubricated condom is totally dependant on fluids from the female. If she has a tendency to be dry, a lubricated condom or the use of a separate lubricant such as Today™ or K-Y Jelly™ may be essential.

Spermicide

Condom makers add the spermicide Nonoxynol-9 to the lubricant in some brands to increase the effectiveness of condoms in protecting against pregnancy.

Condom companies are very cautious when they talk about spermicide. They emphasize that Nonoxynol-9 decreases the risk of pregnancy by reducing the overall number of active sperm, but they emphasize that the extent of the decreased risk has not been established.

Nonoxynol-9 has also been shown to be effective in killing viruses, including the AIDS virus, in laboratory situations, but the level of effectiveness in actual use is not known (see Section #8).

Materials

Today, most condoms are made of latex, although some are still made from animal membrane. Latex condoms are described in Section #16.

Membrane condoms, sometimes called "skins," are considerably more expensive than latex condoms, partly because the supply of membranes, obtained from sheep intestine, is limited. In addition, production costs are higher.

Some people prefer "skins" because they think they are more natural and increase sensitivity. Although membranes may transmit body heat (a key factor in sexual pleasure) better than latex, the difference may be slight, particularly with the thinnest latex condoms, which have a thickness of only .03 mm.

Research indicates that "skins" do not provide the same degree of protection against pregnancy and disease as latex.

To date, latex and animal membrane condoms are the only varieties commercially available, although in the late 1960s a manufacturer of plastic molding machines expressed an interest in selling his machines to establish condom factories in Third World nations.

The manufacturer provided a quantity of plastic condoms to demonstrate the capability of his machines, and the condoms were informally tested. They had an unacceptably high rupture rate, particularly when used by uncircumcised men who had intercourse with the foreskin pulled back to expose the glans.

The plastic from which these condoms were made did not have the elastic properties of latex, which may have contributed to the high breakage rate. Plastics with a wide range of properties are now available and some may be suitable for condoms, although at the time of this writing none are available.

#16 Standards

Latex Condom Classifications

The American Society for Testing and Materials (ASTM) has established standards for latex rubber condoms which cover virtually every aspect of their manufacture, including:

- Their proper construction
- The materials from which they are made
- The testing of individual condoms and batch-sample testing
- Packaging
- Storage and shelf-life

SURFACE: Latex condoms may have two kinds of surface (see Section #15). These are:

- Type I — Smooth surface
- Type II — Textured surface

Maximum weight permitted for Type I condoms is 1.7 g. For Type II, it is 2.0 g.

SHAPE: Latex condoms may have three basic shapes. These are:

- Style 1 — Round end (no tip)
- Style 2 — Reservoir end
- Style 3 — Form-fitting

The reservoir is provided to trap seminal fluid (see Section #15). Style 1 and Style 2 condoms are basically straight in shape. Style 3 condoms are contoured (shaped near the closed end to fit the penis head). The maximum width in this area is 70 mm (2.75 inches) for Class A and 62 mm (2.4 inches) for Class B condoms.

SIZE: There are two basic sizes of latex condoms. These are:

- Class A — 180 mm or 7.1 inches ($\pm$ 20 mm or 0.8 inches) in length and 52 mm or 2.0 inches ($\pm$ 2 mm 0.08 inches) in width
- Class B — 160 mm or 6.3 inches ($\pm$ 10 mm or 0.39 inches) in length and 49 mm or 1.9 inches ($\pm$ 2 mm or 0.08 inches) in width

The thickness of the latex must be between 0.03 and 0.09 mm (0.0012 and .0035 inches).

Each condom packet or multi-packet package of condoms must be legibly marked to show the name or trademark of the manufacturer as well as the date of manufacture, either in coded form or explicitly stated.

Condoms may come in a variety of shades, including:

- Transparent
- Opaque
- Colored

Quality Control

All condoms are individually tested at the time of manufacture to check for defects. The test usually consists of stretching the condom over a frame and then attempting to pass an electric current through it.

Since latex will not conduct electricity, the electric current will pass through the condom only if there are holes in it.

In addition, samples of condom batches are subjected to a series of tests that include filling a condom with three liters of water to check for leakage. The results of these tests are used to calibrate manufacturing processes.

Animal Membrane Condoms

Animal membrane condoms, or "skins," are packaged both rolled and flat. They are packaged with a fluid designed to prevent the membrane from drying out and to serve as a lubricant during intercourse.

Some come in hard plastic capsules; others in foil.

"Skins" do not have tips. They do not cling to the penis as rubber condoms do. They also do not conform to standard sizes for latex condoms, particularly in width.

Two were examined for this book.

One was 180 mm or 7.1 inches long (the same length as Class A latex condoms) and 63 mm or 2.5 inches in width (11 mm or .43 inches wider than Class A latex condoms). The second was 160 mm or 6.3 inches long (the same as Class B latex condoms) and 80 mm or 3.15 inches in width (31 mm or 1.22 inches wider than Class B latex condoms).

To prevent slippage or leakage of fluids, there are elastic bands around the rim to hold the condom onto the penis.

Notes

#17 Sizes

The Need for Different Condom Sizes

Sex therapists say penis size is unimportant in love making; big does not mean better. Penis size may be relevant, however, in choosing a proper-sized condom: a condom that is too small may feel uncomfortably tight, while a condom that is too loose may slip off or allow body fluids to seep in or out.

Measured American Penis Sizes

The pioneer sexologist Kinsey collected data on penis sizes from participants in his studies during the period 1938 to 1963. Kinsey's men were instructed to measure penis length on the top surface from the belly and penis circumference at the maximum point. Measurements were to be to the nearest quarter inch.

Kinsey's subjects were unable to take accurate measurements to the quarter inch, as is evident from his raw data, a sample of which is presented in Table 4. (Note that more men reported penis size at whole - and half-inch marks than at quarter- and three-quarter inch marks.)

The median length of erect penises for white American men (both college and non-college) was 5.9 inches (150 millimeters). That is a statistician's way of saying that half the men had penises less than 5.9 inches long and half had penises longer than 5.9 inches.

Kinsey's data indicate that black American college men (data for black non-college men were not found) have penises that average about a quarter-inch longer than those of white men.

Half of the men in Kinsey's study had penises that measure, when erect, between 5.5 and 6.5 inches (140 and 165 mm) in length.

The median erect penis measured 4.6 inches (117 mm) in circumference. Well over half were between 4.0 and 5.0 inches (102 and 127 mm) in circumference (Ref 8).

Penis Sizes among Asian Men

When the United States Government began supplying condoms to developing nations as part of its international population program, American condoms proved to be too large for many Asian men. A study of penis sizes in Thailand confirmed the difference: Thai men have penises averaging 25 millimeters (one inch) shorter than those of American men (Ref 21).

Deciding What Sizes of Condoms to Make

Medical literature reports erect penises as short as 90 millimeters (3.5 inches) and as long as 330 millimeters (13 inches) (Ref 23). Even these widely varying figures may not represent the biological limits.

It is neither economical nor necessary for condom makers to produce the multiplicity of sizes that might be indicated by the nearly 10 inch (254 mm) difference in penis length reported in the medical literature or the 5.5 inch (140 mm) range in both length and circumference in Kinsey's data.

Ideally, condoms should be long enough to cover the entire penis, but at a minimum the part that comes into contact with the vagina should be covered.

A condom that clings to the penis should do a better job of preventing seepage of body fluids than a loose fitting condom, so, ideally, condoms should be stretched somewhat when worn.

The likelihood of breakage as a result of being stretched over a large penis is probably minimal. One of the standard requirements during quality control tests is that a condom be able to stretch to contain three liters of water without bursting (see Section#16). There is little probability that a man would have a penis mass of even one liter.

Only five percent of Kinsey's subjects would stretch a Class A condom to more than 1.5 times its circumference. Another 25 percent would stretch it from 1.25 to 1.5 times its circumference. Condom companies promote the smaller Class B condoms as being "snugger" rather than smaller, since even larger-sized men could conceivably choose to use them without serious danger of stretching them past the breaking point.

A greater problem may arise with the approximately 15 percent of men with penises smaller than class B condoms.

Condom Marketing and Advertising

Condom companies have a marketing problem. If they make a range of condom sizes and assign names like small, medium and large, customers may be loath to buy those marked small and medium. Informing prospective customers of the existence of a range of condom sizes and styles and how to determine the appropriate product may need to be resolved before additional varieties are offered.

Condom displays in stores generally provide only one level of advertising. Brightly-colored packages tout "enhanced sensitivity" resulting from special lubricants, textured surfaces, form-fitting shape, and ultra-thin latex.

Some brands appeal to female buyers. Women bought about 15 percent of the condoms sold in the mid-1970s. By 1985, they were buying about 40 percent (Ref 24).

Until recently, condom companies had limited opportunities to advertise. Most television stations would not accept condom ads, and in the print media, they were rare except in sex magazines. The AIDS pandemic is changing that.

As condom companies gain more experience with advertising and open marketing, they may well find that a wider range of sizes and their promotion may make economic sense.

#18 Storage

Storage Variables

It is important that condom storage should meet certain requirements. Condoms should be stored:

- At room temperature
- In a dry place
- In a convenient, accessible place
- In their original, unbroken, sealed packet

Exposure to extremes of heat and cold over long periods of time may cause latex as well as lubricants and spermicides to deteriorate. That includes the glove compartment of a car and a wallet carried in a trousers pocket.

A condom carried in the back pocket is subject to friction associated with sitting and walking as well as to body heat.

A fresh condom placed in the front pocket of a jacket is likely to insure the availability of a reliable condom should the need arise.

Moisture may also cause latex to deteriorate. Although the foil wrapping for individual condoms is air- and water-tight when the condom is put into it at the factory, prolonged exposure to water may damage the foil and expose the latex to moisture and air. A damaged package may also admit bacteria.

Condoms should not be removed from the sealed foil until they are to be used. If the seal is discovered to have been broken, the condom should not be used.

Expiration Date

Packages containing condoms with spermicide are labeled with an expiration date for the spermicide.

All condoms or packages of condoms must indicate the manufacturer and date of manufacture. The date may be written on the package in standard, open form or it may be written in a coded form users may not be able to decipher.

Although the manufacturer's identification and expiration dating may be on the package, they are not necessarily easy to read. Dates on some brands are embossed on multicolored or reflective packages but not inked.

Steps in Removing Condoms From Storage

Condoms are generally sealed individually in plastic or foil strips. Care should be taken in opening the package and removing the condom. Tearing off the corner of the foil wrapping to gain access to the condom is preferable to tearing the package across the middle. Fingernails can scratch or poke holes in the latex if the condom is handled too roughly.

Condoms are individually tested at the factory. Further testing is not only unnecessary, it can damage the condom. Blowing the condom up like a balloon can cause weak spots to develop from over-stretching the latex.

#19 Condoms on the Market

Data Collection Procedures

The condoms used for the preparation of this book were purchased in two areas:

- Dallas, TX
- Washington, DC

Price data were collected in five areas:

- Dallas, TX
- Hartford, CT
- Pittsburgh, PA
- San Mateo, CA
- Washington, DC

In addition, the condom marketers were asked for complete lists of brands and styles they market and for samples of their products. Table 7 lists characteristics and prices of condom brands.

The brands listed in Table 7 do not include all those available for sale in the American market, although the brands listed account for an overwhelming majority of recent condom sales.

Some newcomers reportedly have or will shortly enter the market, mostly selling imported condoms.

Class A Condoms

All the latex condoms examined for this book except Trojans had tips or reservoirs to trap seminal fluid.

Trojans are plain, round-end, no frills con-doms.
(Carter-Wallace, maker of Trojan, markets a full line of condoms using names like Trojan Ribbed, Trojan Plus, etc. See below.)

Unlubricated Class A Condoms

All but two brands of Class A condoms were lubricated. The unlubricated brands are Trojans and Trojan-Enz.

Trojan-Enz are available either lubricated or dry.

Class A Condoms with Spermicide

The lubricant in three brands contained a spermicide:

- Comfort Fit
- Ramses Extra
- Sheik Elite

The Comfort Fit condom was purchased from a vending machine at a truck stop in Texas in May 1987, about a month after the "4/15/87" expiration date for the spermicide.

Form-Fitted Class A Condoms

Four Class A brands were form-fitted or con-toured to the shape of the penis:

- LifeStyle Conture
- Ramses Nuform
- Trojan Plus
- Trojan Naturalube

The Trojan Naturalube was also textured.

Textured Class A Condoms

Four Class A brands were textured but not contoured:

- Excita Fiesta
- Excita Ultra Ribbed
- LifeStyle Stimula
- Trojan Ribbed

The Mentor Contraceptive

The Mentor Contraceptive consists of a condom inside an "applicator hood" that covers approximately half the length of the condom.

The manufacturer claims that this contraceptive is safer than ordinary condoms because of a unique Safety-Seal™ that "prevents the condom from accidentally coming off during use, plus it forms a watertight barrier which keeps fluids from seeping in or out."

The manufacturer emphasizes that the penis must be dry when the device is put on and that no lubricant or spermicide should be put on the penis or condom prior to vaginal entry. Lubricants and spermicide may be used in the vagina before beginning intercourse.

The user unrolls the Mentor condom with hood onto his erect penis. He then squeezes the contraceptive all around the penis shaft to secure the Safety Seal™.

A twisting action removes the hood, a must before vaginal entry.

The package contains detailed instructions on how to use this contraceptive. Given its uniqueness, the instructions are absolutely essential.

The sealed white container for individual contraceptives is considerably thicker than packages containing ordinary condoms.

Mentor Corporation's product lines include surgically-implantable medical devices and disposable medical products. Its unique condom device employs technology from the company's medical products.

Class B Condoms

Table 7 includes three Class B lubricated and form-fitted condoms:

- Protex Secure
- Sheik Fetherlite SnugFit
- Protex Arouse

Unlubricated Secure condoms are also available.

Textured Class B Condoms

The Protex Arouse was the only textured Class B condom found. It has two types of texturing: rings or spirals near the closed end of the condom (near the head of the penis) and nodules - small specks of latex - covering the shaft from the neck to just above the rim.

Animal Membrane Condoms

There were two animal membrane condoms or "skins:"

- Kling-Tite Naturalamb
- Fourex

Animal membrane condoms vary widely in size (see Section #17). The Kling-Tite condom sample was as long as a Class A latex condom - 180 mm long (7.1 inches) - but 63 mm (2.5 inches) wide. The Fourex was the same length as a Class B latex condom - 160 mm long (6.3 inches) - but 80 mm (3.15 inches) wide.

Both are available either rolled or unrolled and both are packaged with a fluid that keeps the "skin" moistened and serves as lubricant.

The texture of animal membrane condoms is different than latex, and animal membrane does not have the elastic properties of latex. To hold the looser-fitting "skins" on and to prevent leakage, there are elastic bands around the rim.

Condom Packaging

Condoms are available in drug stores and supermarkets in three quantities: 3, 12 and 36. Packages containing a single condom (and possibly other quantities) are available in vending machines at truck stops and other places catering to travellers, presumably so they will be available to meet unexpected needs.

Trojan Assortment is a marketing strategy rather than a different condom. The package contains 12 condoms, four each of three different condoms marketed by Carter-Wallace including:

- Trojan-Enz
- Trojan Ribbed
- Trojan Plus

Novelty Condoms

A Korean-made device labeled a "French Tickler" was purchased from a vending machine in a Texas truck stop. It was clearly labeled as a novelty item and the labeling included the warning that it was not intended "for the prevention of disease." French Ticklers have been around for years.

The Tickler appears to be an ordinary non-lubricated condom to which large nodules have been attached. The nodules measured five millimeters. There were six in all, arranged in two rows on opposing sides of the condom near the closed end.

Nodules on ordinary "ribbed" condoms are tiny compared to those on the French Tickler.

The Tickler is probably truly a novelty item, not intended for use in sexual intercourse. It could do serious physical harm.

Condom Prices

Condom prices at the retail level range from as little as 19 cents for Protex Touch priced in Dallas to $2.80 for Fourex natural skins in the District of Columbia. Considering the pattern of prices, the 19-cent Protex Touch, a lubricated condom with a tip, was exceptional.

Probably more typical on the low end of the range was 25 cents for plain, no-frills Trojans and 26 cents for non-lubricated Trojan-Enz, both in Hartford.

Table 6 shows the lowest and highest prices for each brand found by those who price-shopped.

The Mentor Contraceptive and the condoms made of animal membrane were the most expensive. They range from about $1.66 to $2.80.

Price shopping for condoms and purchases of packages containing 12 or 36 condoms can produce considerable savings.

For example, a package containing 36 Trojans in Hartford was priced at $8.85, a unit price of 25 cents. A package of three Trojans cost $1.79 for a unit price of 60 cents in both Hartford and Washington.

Condoms With Carrying Cases

One new twist to condom marketing is the introduction of carrying cases. Two brands were examined: Koromex and LifeStyle Extra Strength. The carrying cases resemble small wallets. The LifeStyle package purchased for this book contained four condoms and a carrying-case measuring, when folded, 3 X 2.75 inches. The Koromex package contained 12 condoms and a case measuring, when folded, 4.75 X 2.63 inches. Both cases are easily carried in a woman's purse, making them appealing to female customers. The cases also easily fit into a man's or woman's jacket.

Both brands have the spermicide, Nonoxynol-9. The LifeStyle brand puts an extra quantity of Nonoxynol-9 in the condom tip.

Other Brands

In response to the expanded interest in condoms and the greater freedom to talk about them, condom makers have introduced a variety of brands with catchy names like Pleaser, Man Form, Embraceher, Sensuals, Kimono and Chapeau Blackey. There will surely be more brands as condom companies respond to concerns about AIDS and to the enhanced respectability of condoms.

A Female Condom

Researchers in England have reported the development of Femshield, a condom for women. Femshield resembles a small plastic bag. It has a large plastic ring at the open end to secure the device to the outside of the vagina and a small ring at the closed end to be placed at the cervix. Femshield is made of polyurethane, a stronger and lighter material than the latex used to make condoms.

Femshield can be inserted well before intercourse. It requires the use of a lubricant inside the condom to prevent penile irritation. Men are said to prefer the female condom because it is not tight like the male device. The device is currently being tested (Ref 26).

The idea for a female condom is not new. Roman legend refers to the use of a goat's bladder as a female condom, but whether the Romans actually used a female condom is not known (see Section #2).

Larger Condoms

Mentor recently introduced a new line of large condoms.

TABLE 1
PERCENT OF REPRODUCTIVE AGE COUPLES USING COITUS INTERRUPTUS: SELECTED COUNTRIES

Country	Percent Using
Bulgaria	60
Italy	36
Yugoslavia	36
Romania	26
Portugal	25
Belgium ★	23
Spain	22
France	21
Poland	19
Hungary	17
Philippines	10

★ Flemish part only.

Reference: 17

TABLE 2
PERCENT OF REPRODUCTIVE AGE COUPLES USING VASECTOMY: SELECTED COUNTRIES

Country	Percent Using
Netherlands	11
United States	10
United Kingdom	8
South Korea	6

Reference: 17

TABLE 3
PERCENT OF REPRODUCTIVE AGE COUPLES USING CONDOMS: SELECTED COUNTRIES

Country or Area	Percent Using
Japan	50
Finland	32
Denmark	25
United Kingdom	18
Trinidad & Tobago	17
Norway	16
Poland	14
Italy	13
Taiwan	12
Netherlands	11
United States ★	10
Costa Rica	9
Switzerland	8
Jamaica	8
Belgium ★ ★	7
Sao Paulo, Brazil	7
Fiji	6
France	6
Korea, South	6
Portugal	6
Surabaya, Indonesia	6
Barbados	5
Semerang, Indonesia	5
Spain	5
Venezuela	5

★ Excludes Alaska & Hawaii   ★ ★ Flemish part only.

Reference: 17

TABLE 4
RAW DATA ON MEASURED PENILE LENGTH FROM KINSEY STUDY

Length in Inches	White College	White non College	Black College
5.50	10.7	8.4	5.1
5.75	8.0	2.8	5.1
6.00	23.9	23.8	25.4
6.25	8.8	10.5	10.2
6:50	14.3	15.4	16.9

Reference: 8

TABLE 5
DIRECT AND INDIRECT SEXUAL PARTNERS

Year	Annual Number of Partners	
	Two	**Three**
This Year	2	3
Last Year	6	12
2 Years Ago	14	39
3 Years Ago	30	120
4 Years Ago	62	363
5 Years Ago	126	1,092
6 Years Ago	264	3,276
Total	504	4,905

TABLE 6
CHARACTERISTICS AND PRICE RANGES
FOR CONDOMS SOLD IN THE UNITED STATES

Characteristic and Brand	Tip	Lub	FF	Tex	SC	Unit Price $	
						Low	High
Class A Condoms							
Trojans	No	No	No	No	No	.25	.60
Trojan-Enz	Yes	No	No	No	No	.26	.36
Excell	Yes	Yes	No	No	No	— .35 —	
LifeStyle Nuda	Yes	Yes	No	No	No	.61	.69
Protex Touch	Yes	Yes	No	No	No	.19	.35
Ramses Sensitol	Yes	Yes	No	No	No	.48	1.05
Trojan-Enz	Yes	Yes	No	No	No	.36	.70
LifeStyle Conture	Yes	Yes	Yes	No	No	n/a	n/a
Ramses Nuform	Yes	Yes	Yes	No	No	.37	.75
Trojan Plus	Yes	Yes	Yes	No	No	.36	.50
Trojan Naturalube	Yes	Yes	Yes	Yes	No	.30	.62
Excita Fiesta	Yes	Yes	No	Yes	No	.35	.57
Excita Ultra Ribbed	Yes	Yes	No	Yes	No	.36	.50
LifeStyle Stimula	Yes	Yes	No	Yes	No	.58	.73

	Tip	Lub	FF	Tex	SC		
Trojan Ribbed	Yes	Yes	No	Yes	No	.39	.82
Comfort Fit	Yes	Yes	No	No	Yes	n/a	n/a
Ramses Extra	Yes	Yes	No	No	Yes	— .94 —	
Sheik Elite	Yes	Yes	No	No	Yes	.37	.50
Mentor Contraceptive		(see Section #20)				1.66	2.00
Class B Condoms							
Protex Secure	Yes	Yes	Yes	No	No	— .52 —	
Shell Fetherlite	Yes	Yes	Yes	No	No	.36	.66
Protex Arouse	Yes	Yes	Yes	Yes	No	.38	.51
Membrane Condoms							
Fourex	No	Yes	No	No	No	1.74	2.80
Kling-Tite	No	Yes	No	No	No	1.67	2.45

Key:

	Meaning
Tip	Reservoir Tip
Lub	Lubricated
FF	Form Fitted
Tex	Textured Surface
SC	Spermicide

TABLE 7

CONDOMS PROVIDED BY USAID TO SELECTED AFRICAN NATIONS: 1984 TO 1989

Country	Annual Shipments					
	1984	1985	1986	1987	1988	1989 *
	Condoms (units)					
Botswana	1,410,000	678,000	1,170,000	2,076,000	4,494,000	1,206,000
Burundi	0	6,000	0	300,000	0	0
Ghana	828,000	4,422,000	2,010,000	1,662,000	9,102,000	3,018,000
Kenya	306,500	454,300	6,306,000	12,300,000	13,332,000	18,894,000
Senegal	715,000	1,098,000	24,000	756,000	606,000	2,550,000
Togo	24,000	390,000	18,000	372,000	2,004,000	522,000
Uganda	1,076,400	336,000	318,000	2,250,000	5,844,000	3,288,000
Zimbabwe	1,002,000	8,046,000	3,168,000	10,536,000	10,974,000	10,014,000
Total	5,361,900	15,430,300	13,014,000	30,252,000	46,356,000	39,492,000

*Information provided through September

Notes

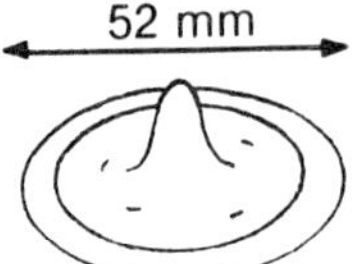

Rolled Condom

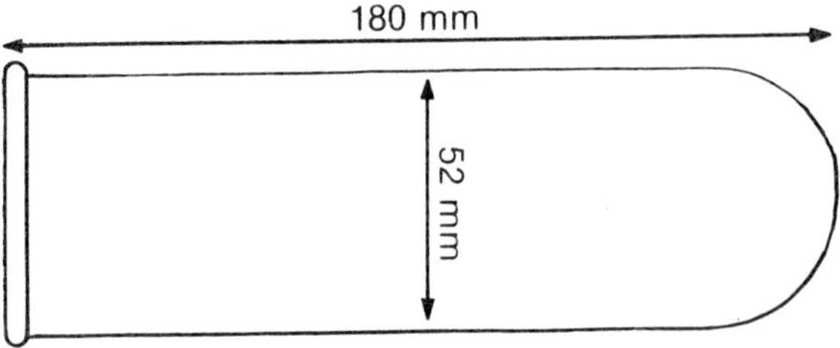

Round End Condom

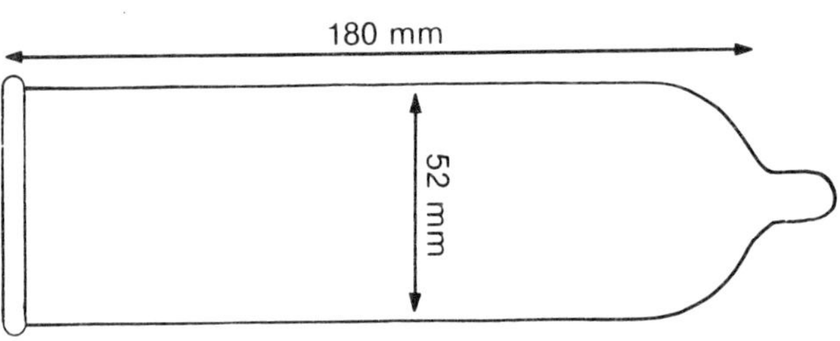

Tipped Condom

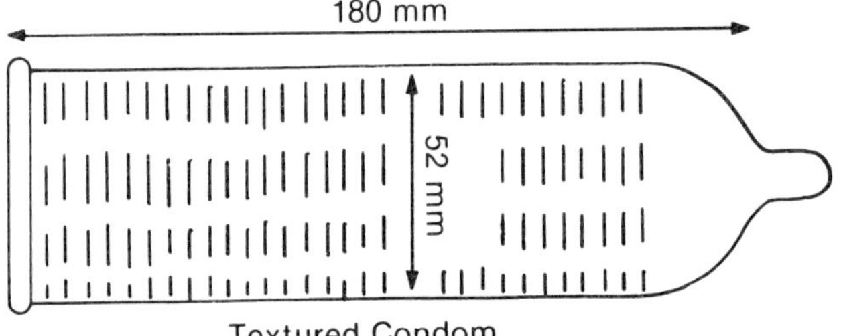

Textured Condom

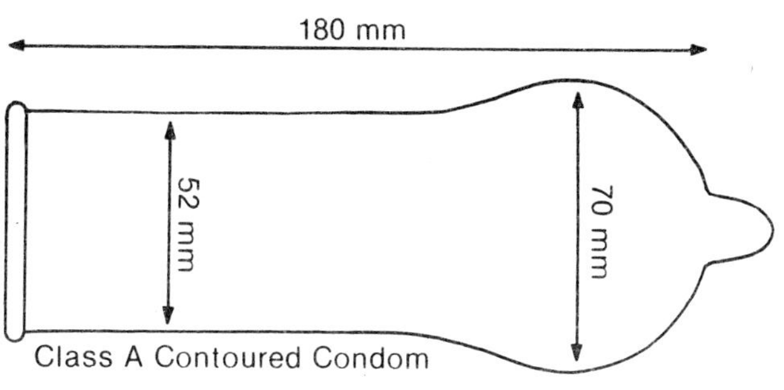

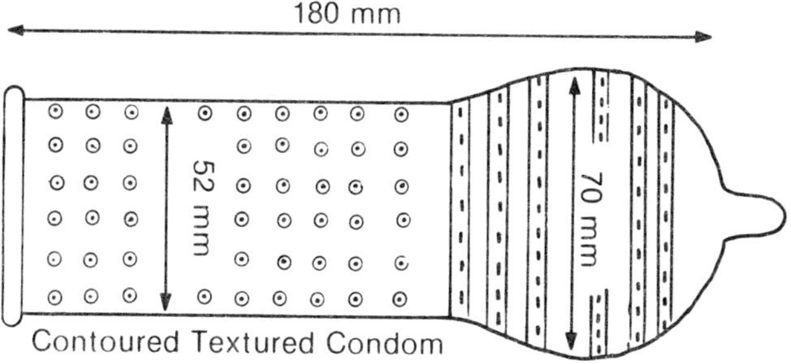

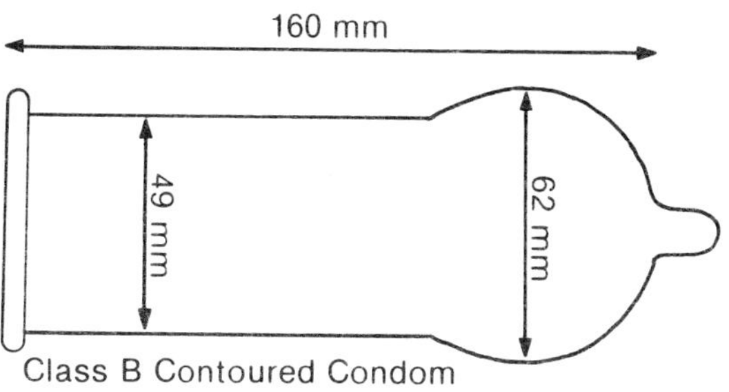

21.

Note that the rolled, extra latex material is always on the outside

References

1.   Conant M, et al: Condoms prevent transmission of AIDS-associated retrovirus (letter). JAMA 1986;255(13):1706.

2.   Conant MA, Spicer DW, Smith CD: Herpes simplex virus transmission: condom study. Sexually Transmitted Diseases 1984;11(2):94-5.

3.   Connell EB, Tatum HJ: Reproductive Health Care Manual (2nd ed.) Durant, OK: Creative Infomatics, Inc., 1986.

4.   Connell EB, Tatum HJ: Sexually Transmitted Diseases. Durant, OK: Creative Infomatics, Inc., 1986.

5.   Coram R: Rubbers from Ronnie. Playboy, 1987;6:36.

6.   Craske J: HTLV-3 infection and AIDS: Risk of spread by heterosexual contact. IPPF Medical Bulletin 1986;20(1):3-4.

7.   Des Larlais DC, et al: HTLV-III/LAV transmission and 'safer' sexual practices in Rwanda and New York City [abstract]. In: International Symposium on African AIDS, Brussels 22-23 Nov 1985, Program and Abstracts [Unpublished].

8.   Gebhard PH, Johnson AB: The Kinsey Data: Marginal Tabulations of the 1938-1963 Interviews Conducted by the Institute for Sex-Research. Philadelphia, PA: W. B. Saunders Company, 1979.

9.   Gruson L: Condoms: Experts fear false sense of security. New York Times, August 18, 1987.

10.   Haeberle EJ: The Sex Atlas, A New Illustrated Guide. New York:The Seabury Press, 1978.

11.   Hines NE: Medical History of Contraception. New York: Gamut Press,1936 and 1963.

12.   Jacobs G, Kerrins J: The AIDS File. Woods Hole, MA: Cromlech Books, Inc., 1987.

13.   Katsnelson S, Drew WL, Mintz L: Efficacy of the condom as a barrier to the transmission of cytomegalovirus. Journal of Infectious Diseases 1984;150:155-7.

14.   Kish LS, et al: An ancient method and a modern scourge: the condom as a barrier against herpes (letter). Journal of the American Academy of Dermatology 1983;9(5):769-70.

15.   Minuk GY, Bohme CE, Bowen TJ: Condoms and hepatitis B virus infection (letter). Annals of Internal Medicine1986;104(4):584.

16.   Pechter K: The great condom test of 1986. Men's Health 1986.

17. Population Information Program: Fertility and family planning surveys: an update. Population Reports, Series M, Number 8, September-October 1985.

18. Remis R: When may a couple stop using condoms? JAMA1987;257(17)

19. Shenfelt PD: The condom as a contraceptive and prophylactic — an appraisal. Wisconsin Medical Journal, 1982;80(9):19-20. Citedin: Population Reports: Update on condoms — products, protection, promotion. Series H, Number 6, September-October 1982.

20. Test confirms condoms block AIDS virus. Medical World News 1986;27(2):32-32.

21. The Johns Hopkins University Population Information Program: Update on condoms — products, protection, promotion. Population Reports, Series H, Number 6, September-October 1982.

22. Waites G: Improving male methods. World Health Organization, Special Programme of Research, Development and Research Training in Human Reproduction. People 1986;1(13):5-6.

23. Wanderer Z, Radell D: The Book of Sexual Measurements: How Big is Big? New York: Bell Publishing Company, 1982.

24. Wilkinson S: Selling condoms to women: liberation plus legislation gives new life to the old rubber. Working Woman 1985:10.

25. Winkelstein W Jr., et al: The San Francisco Men's Health Study:III. Reduction in human immunodeficiency virus transmission among homosexual/bisexual men, 1982-86. American Journal of Public Health 1987;6.

26. The Alan Guttmacher Institute: A female condom? Fam Plan Perspec 1988;20(3).

27. Consumer Reports: Can you rely on condoms? March, 1989.

28. Brackett JW, Demand for and accessibility to family planning services in Subsaharan Africa. Report prepared under contract with the Africa Bureau of the United States Agency for International Development, October, 1989.